Y0-CVK-035

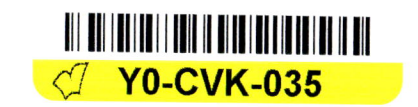

Kansas City, MO Public Library
0000188970792

LET'S LOOK AT BODY SYSTEMS!

DAX'S DEPENDABLE DIGESTIVE SYSTEM

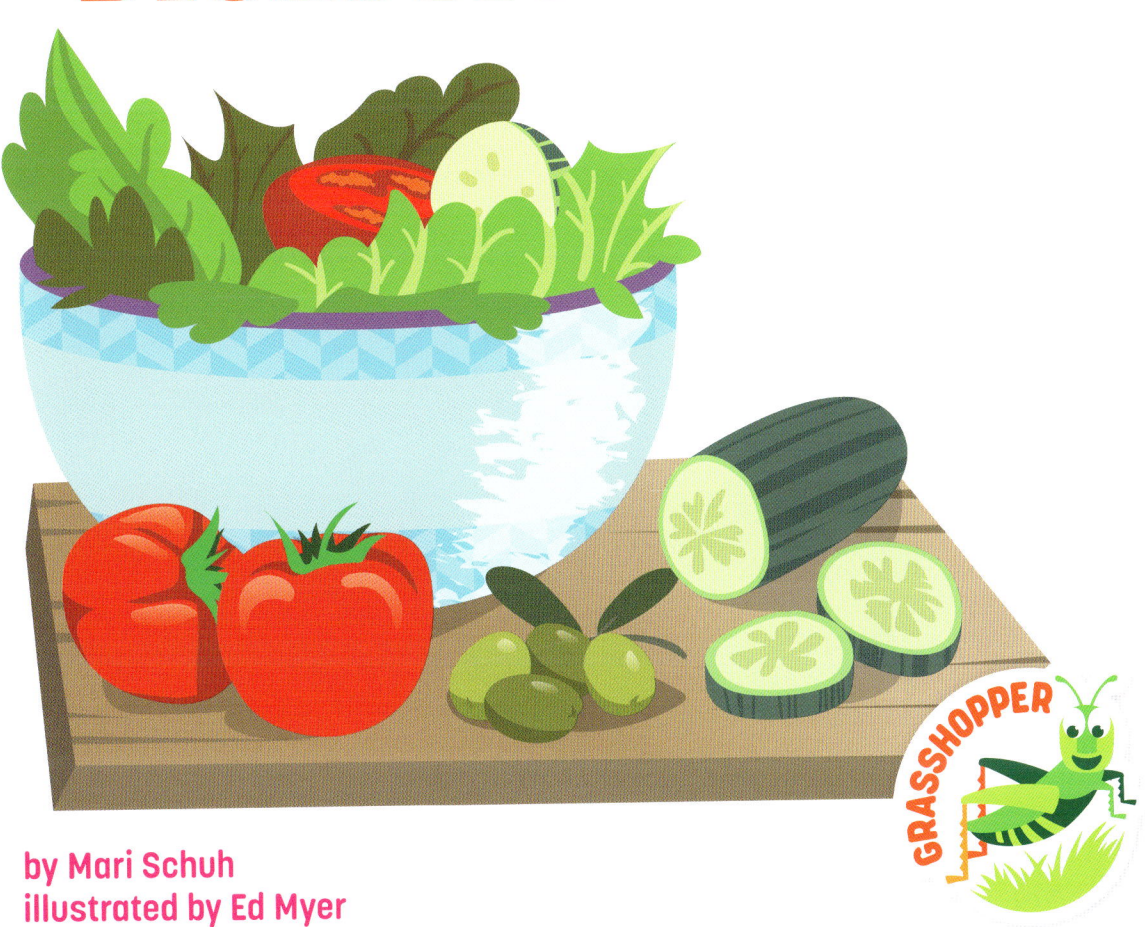

by Mari Schuh
illustrated by Ed Myer

GRASSHOPPER

Tools for Parents & Teachers

Grasshopper Books enhance imagination and introduce the earliest readers to fiction with fun storylines and illustrations. The easy-to-read text supports early reading experiences with repetitive sentence patterns and sight words.

Before Reading

- Discuss the cover illustration. What do they see?
- Look at the glossary together. Discuss the words.

Read the Book

- Read the book to the child, or have him or her read independently.
- "Walk" through the book and look at the illustrations. Who is the main character? What is happening in the story?

After Reading

- Prompt the child to think more. Ask: Think about the food you eat each day. How does your digestive system turn it into energy?

Grasshopper Books are published by Jump!
5357 Penn Avenue South
Minneapolis, MN 55419
www.jumplibrary.com

Copyright © 2022 Jump! International copyright reserved in all countries. No part of this book may be reproduced in any form without written permission from the publisher.

Library of Congress Cataloging-in-Publication Data

Names: Schuh, Mari C., 1975- author. | Myer, Ed, illustrator.
Title: Dax's dependable digestive system / by Mari Schuh; illustrated by Ed Myer.
Description: Minneapolis, MN: Jump!, Inc., [2022]
Series: Let's look at body systems! | Includes index.
Audience: Ages 7-10
Identifiers: LCCN 2021038009 (print)
LCCN 2021038010 (ebook)
ISBN 9781636906386 (hardcover)
ISBN 9781636906393 (paperback)
ISBN 9781636906409 (ebook)
Subjects: LCSH: Digestive organs–Juvenile literature.
Digestion–Juvenile literature.
Classification: LCC QP145 .S32 2022 (print)
LCC QP145 (ebook) | DDC 612.3–dc23
LC record available at https://lccn.loc.gov/2021038009
LC ebook record available at https://lccn.loc.gov/2021038010

Editor: Jenna Gleisner
Direction and Layout: Anna Peterson
Illustrator: Ed Myer

Printed in the United States of America at Corporate Graphics in North Mankato, Minnesota.

Table of Contents

Food on the Move	4
Where in the Body?	22
Let's Review!	23
To Learn More	23
Glossary	24
Index	24

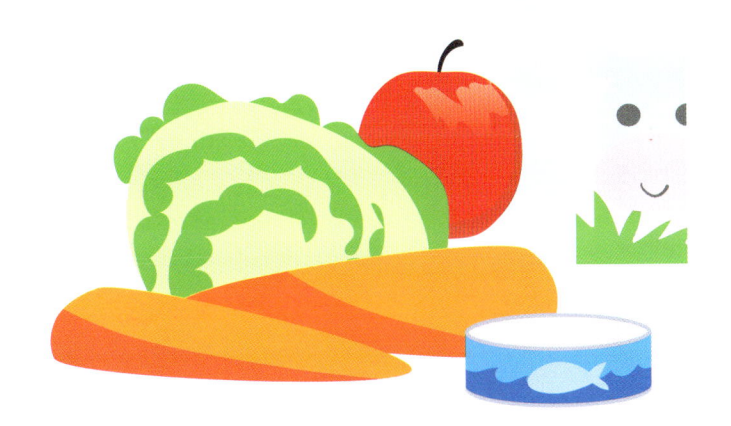

Food on the Move

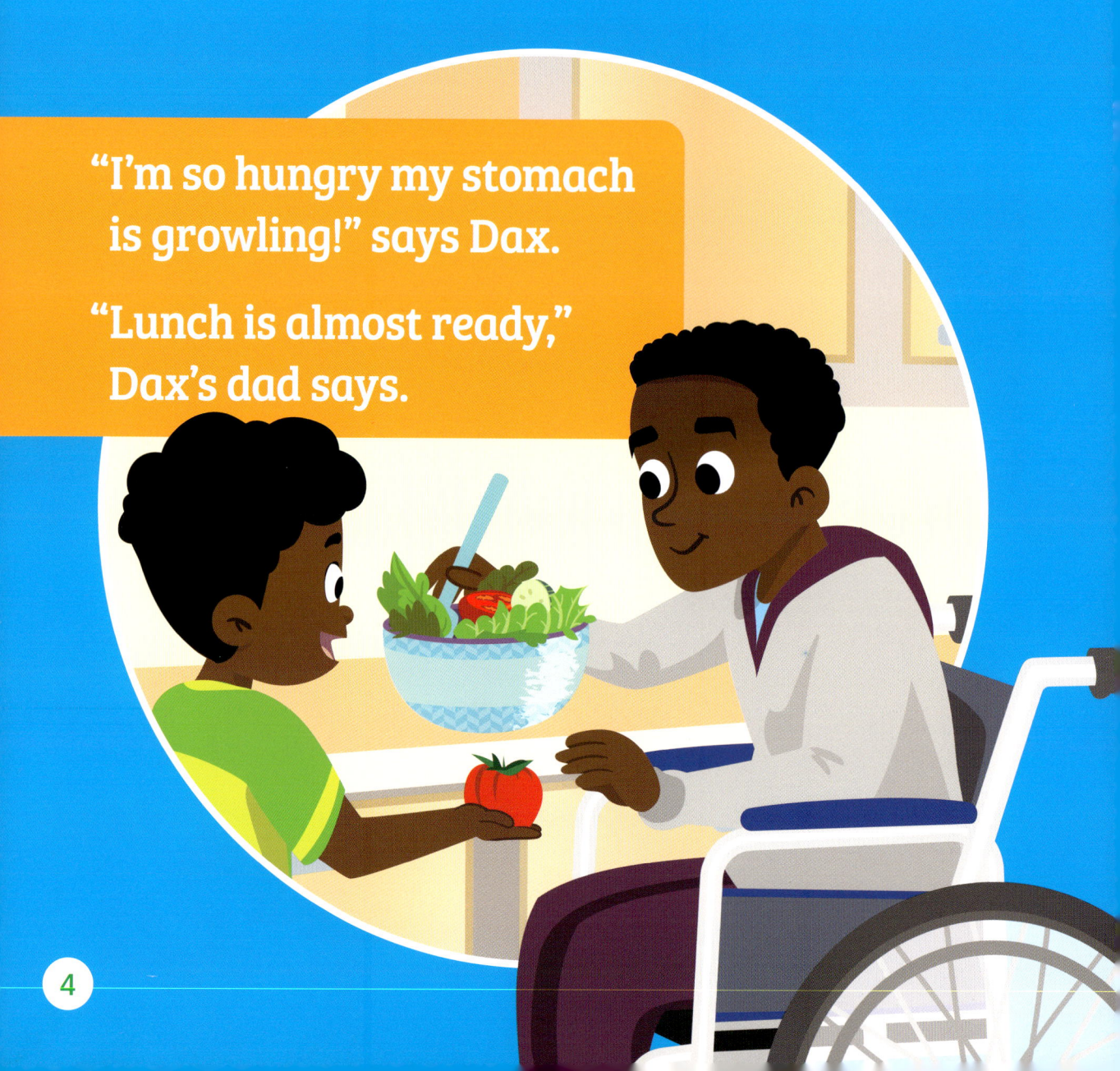

"I'm so hungry my stomach is growling!" says Dax.

"Lunch is almost ready," Dax's dad says.

"What happens to food after I eat it?" Dax asks.

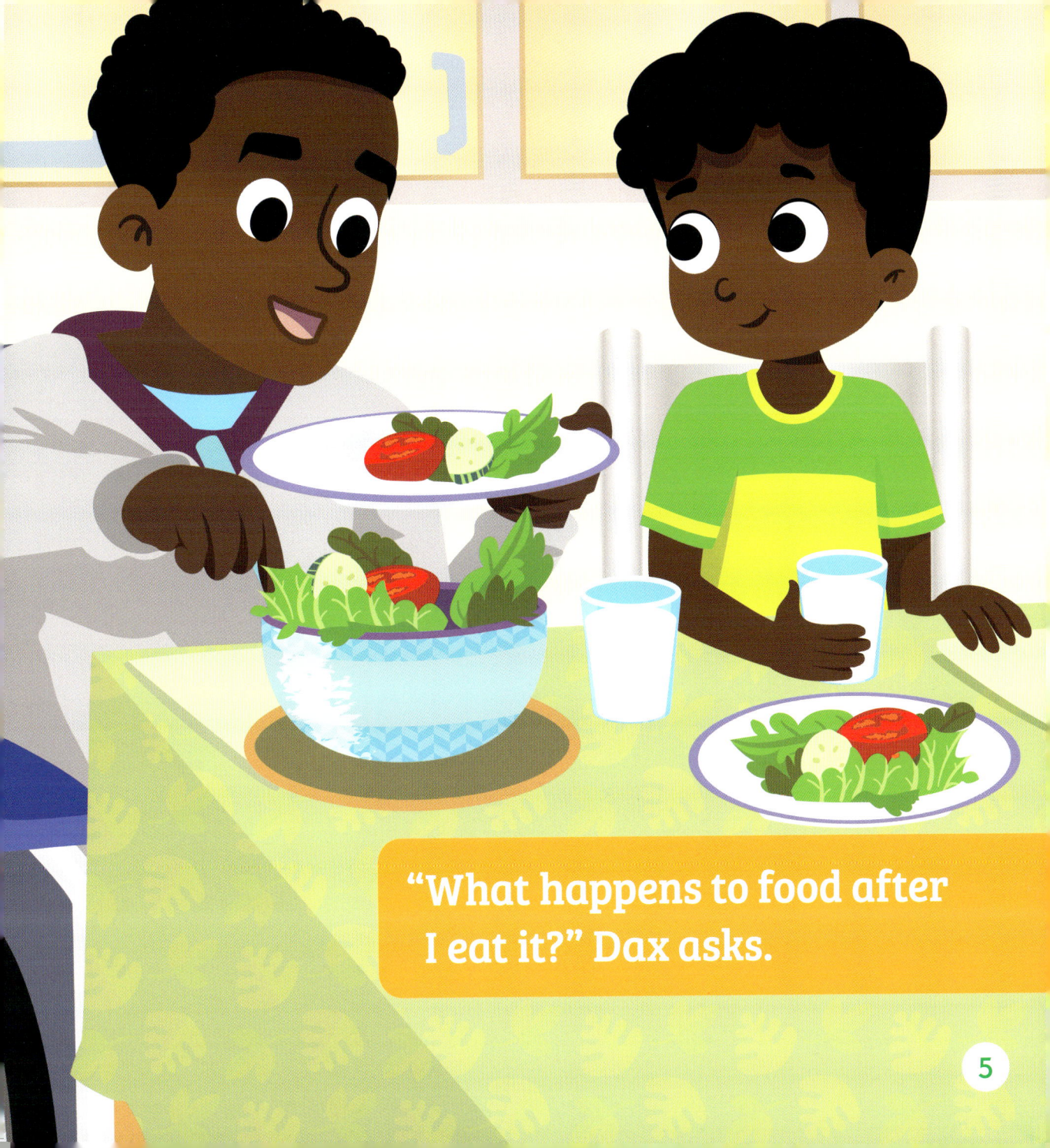

"You digest it! Your body's digestive system turns the foods you eat into nutrients. Then your body uses nutrients for energy. Did you know digestion actually starts with your mouth?" his dad replies.

"Really? How?" Dax asks.

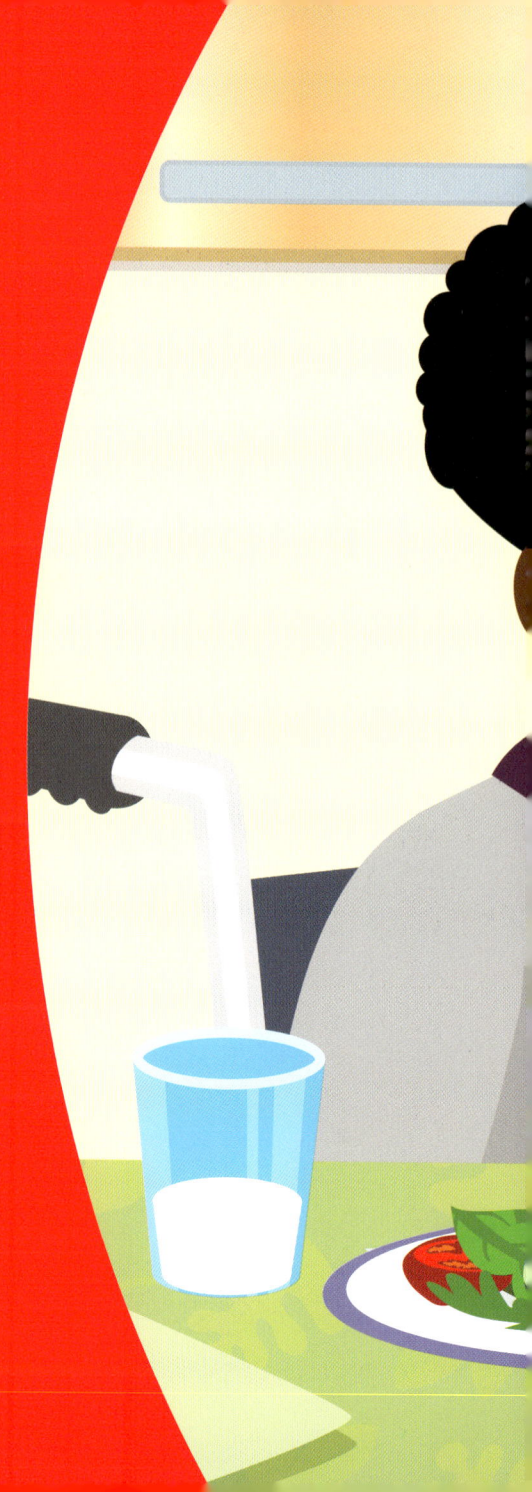

7

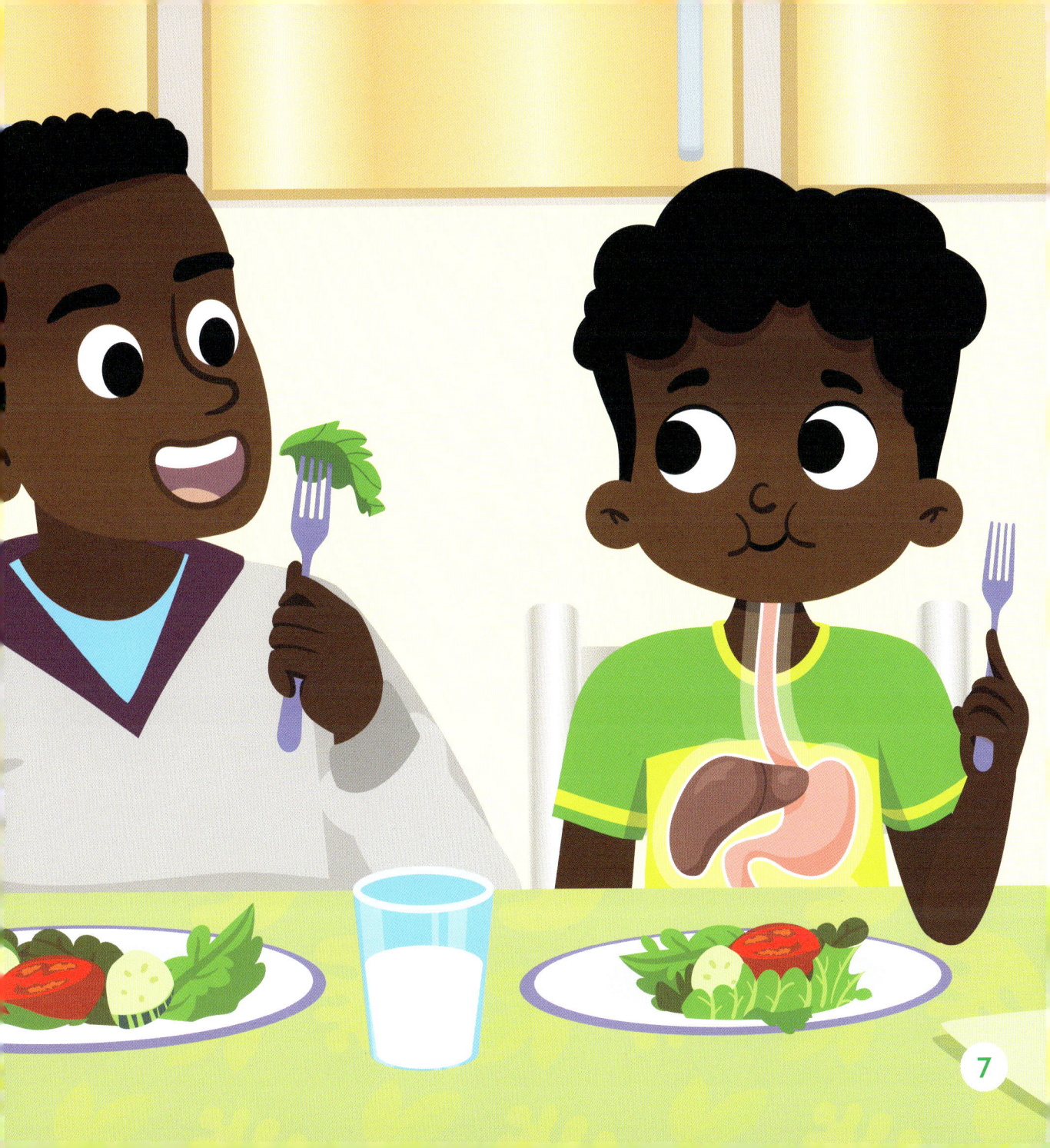

"Your teeth chew and grind the food you eat," Dax's dad says. "Your tongue mixes the food with saliva to make it soft and wet."

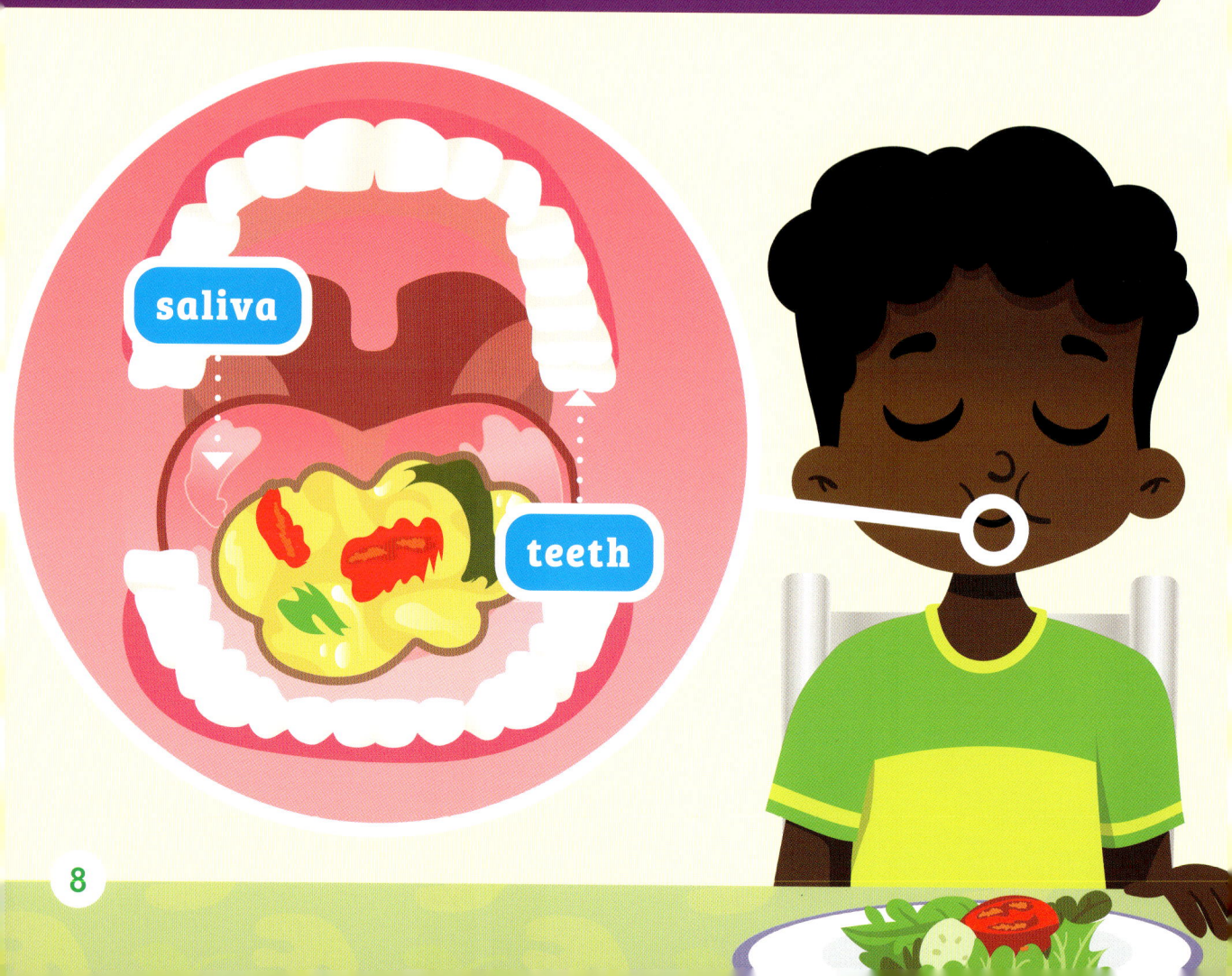

saliva

teeth

esophagus

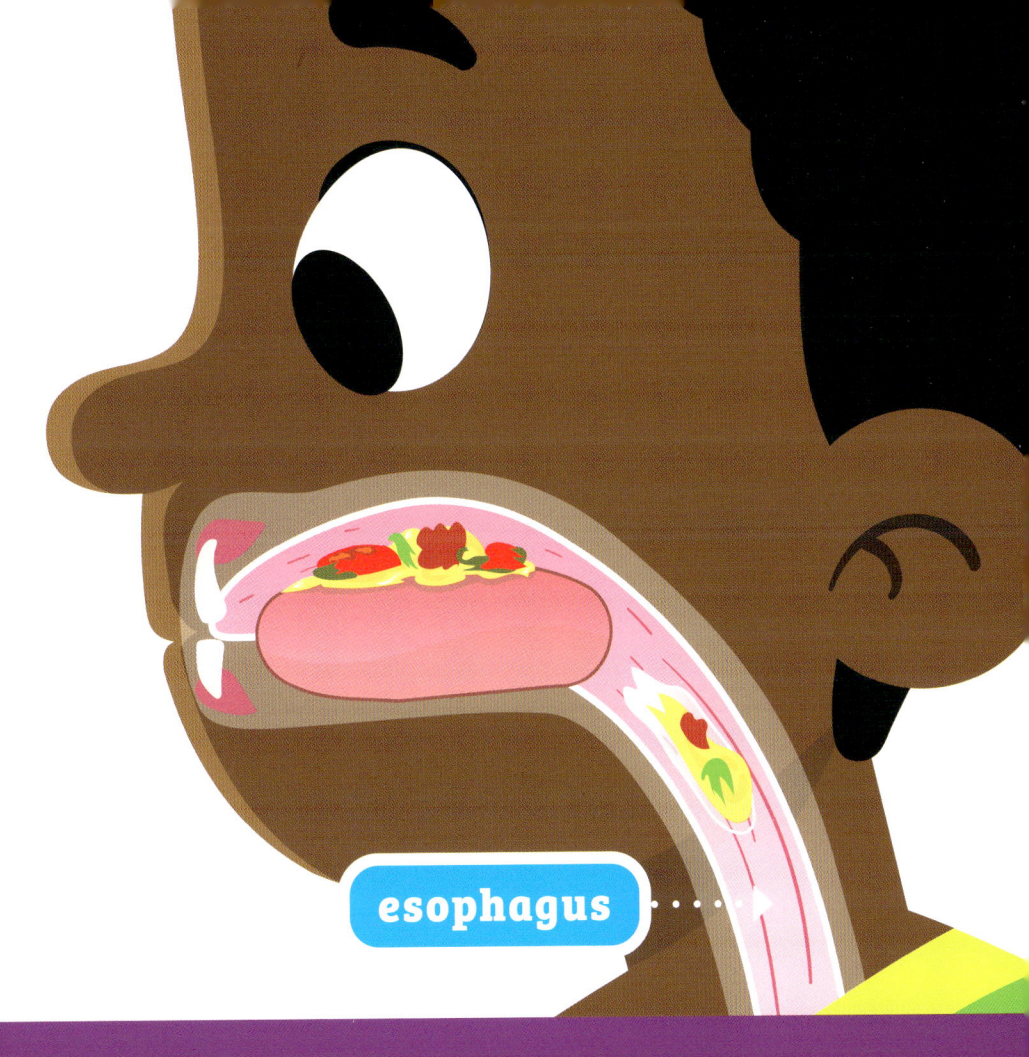

"Then you swallow the food. It goes down a tube called the esophagus and into your stomach," he explains.

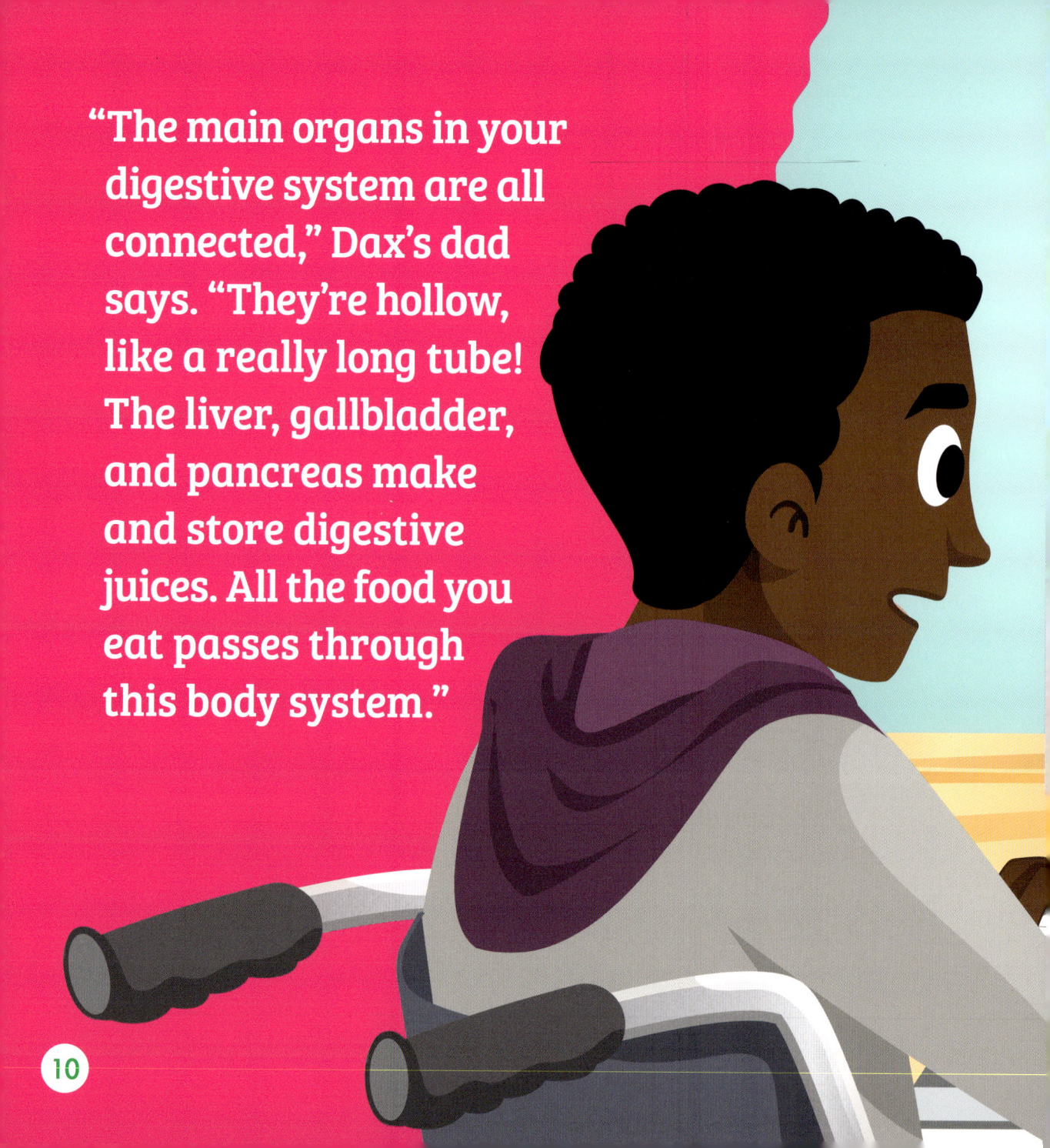

"The main organs in your digestive system are all connected," Dax's dad says. "They're hollow, like a really long tube! The liver, gallbladder, and pancreas make and store digestive juices. All the food you eat passes through this body system."

11

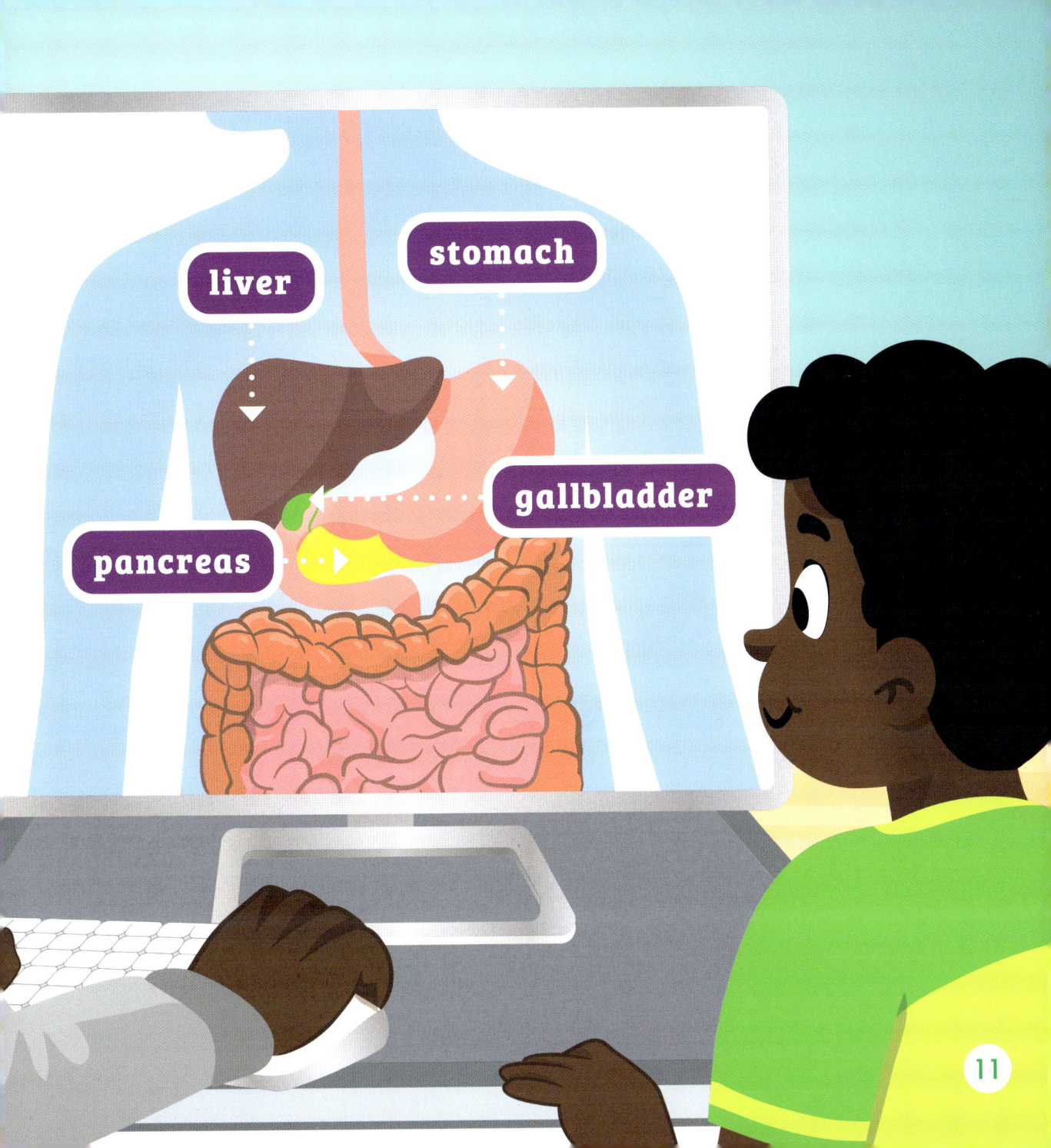

"How does food turn into energy my body can use?" Dax asks.

"Juices in the stomach have acid and enzymes," his dad says. "They mix with the food and break it down into a thick liquid."

stomach

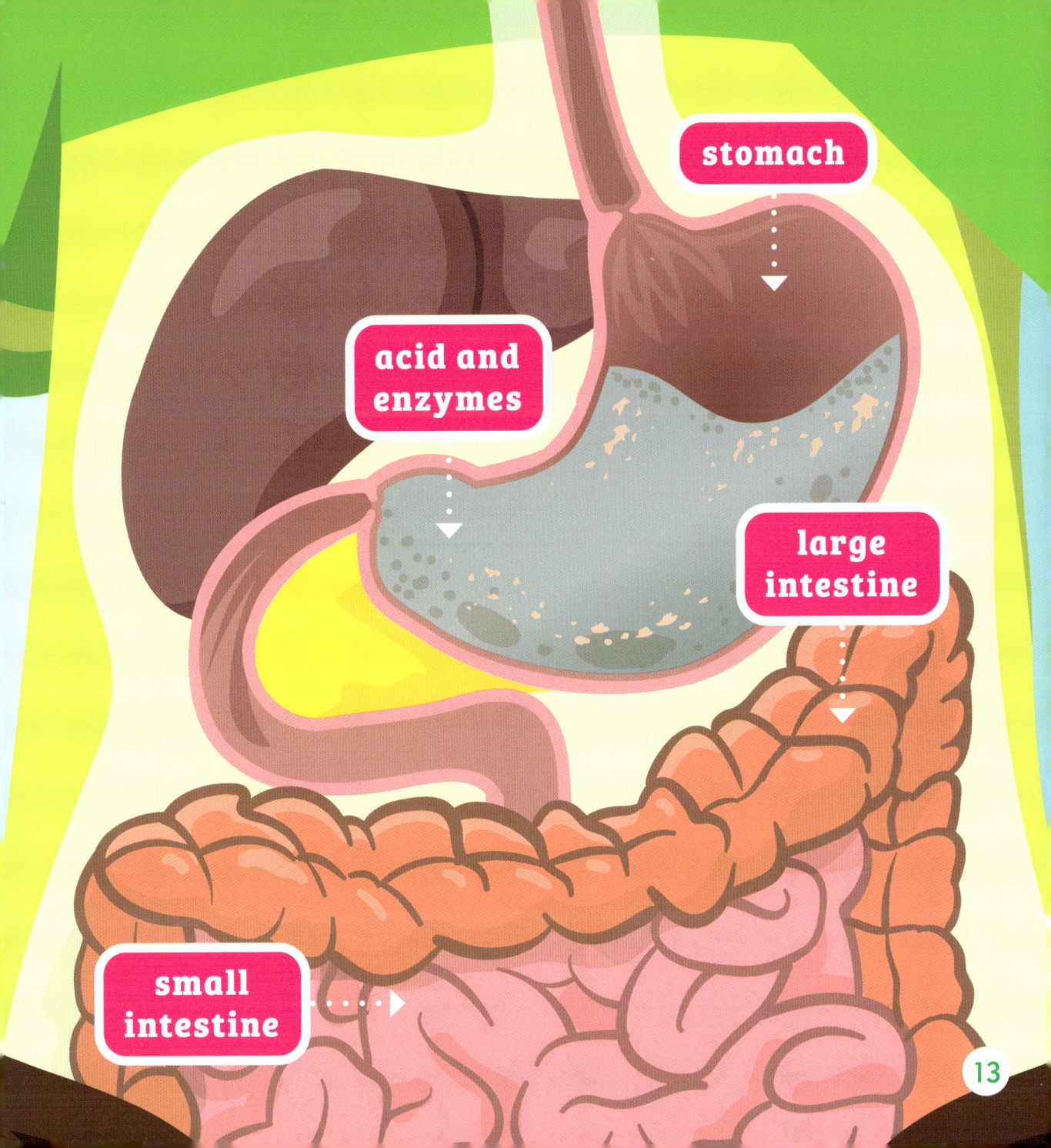

acid and enzymes

large intestine

small intestine

"Nutrients from the liquid go into your blood through the walls of the small intestine. Blood delivers the nutrients to your body's cells. Your cells use the nutrients for energy, to repair tissues, and for growth," his dad says.

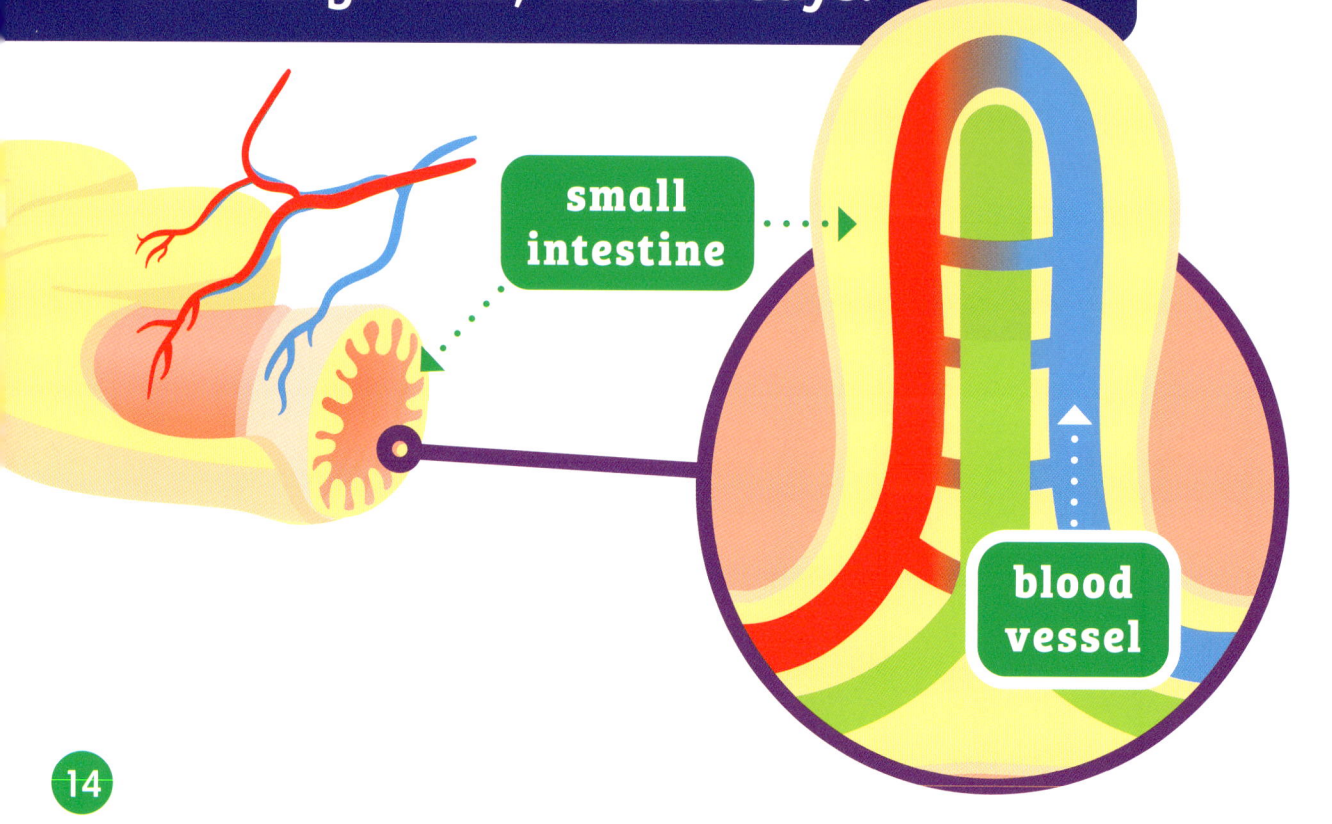

small intestine

blood vessel

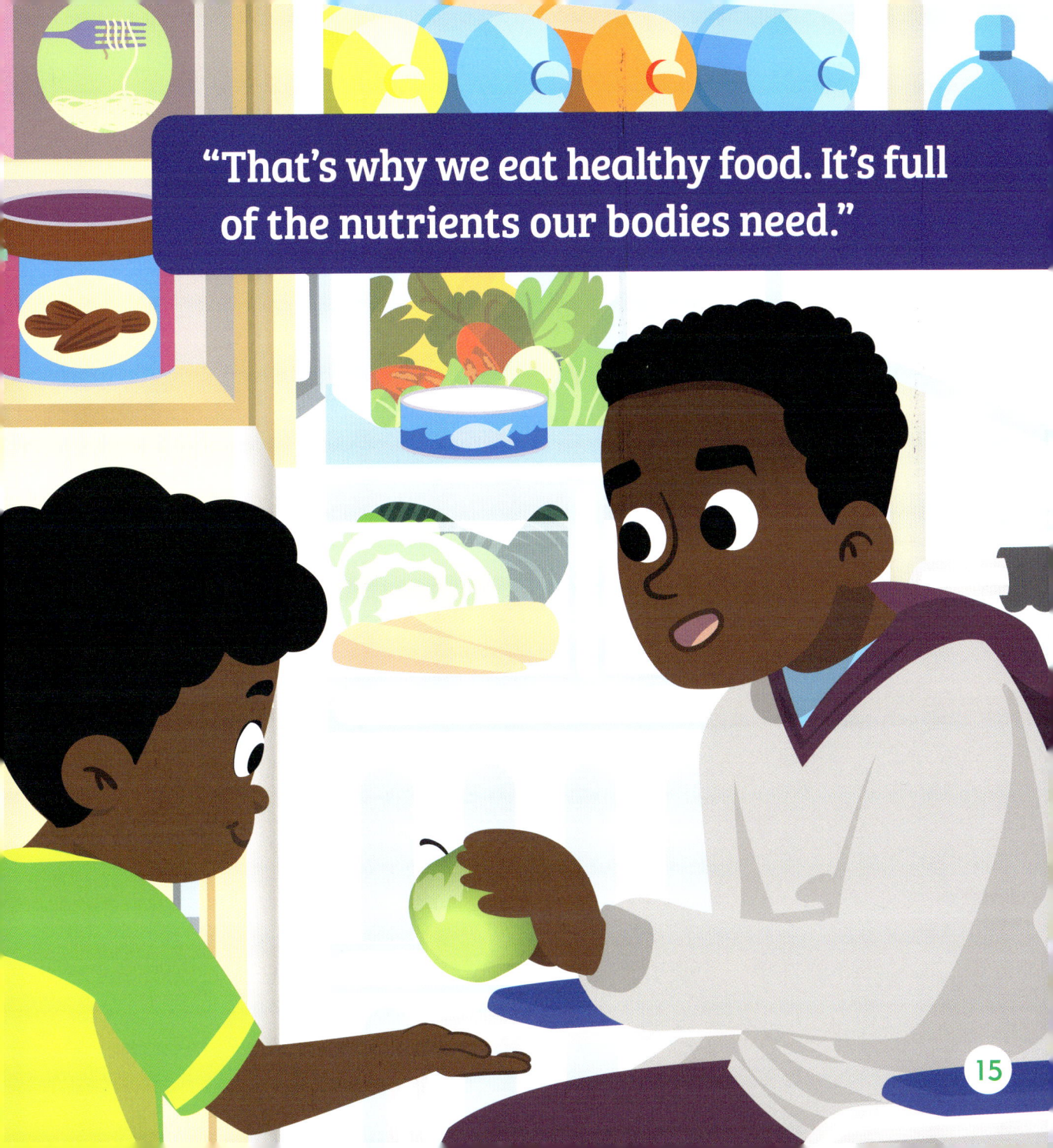

"That's why we eat healthy food. It's full of the nutrients our bodies need."

"What happens next?" Dax asks.

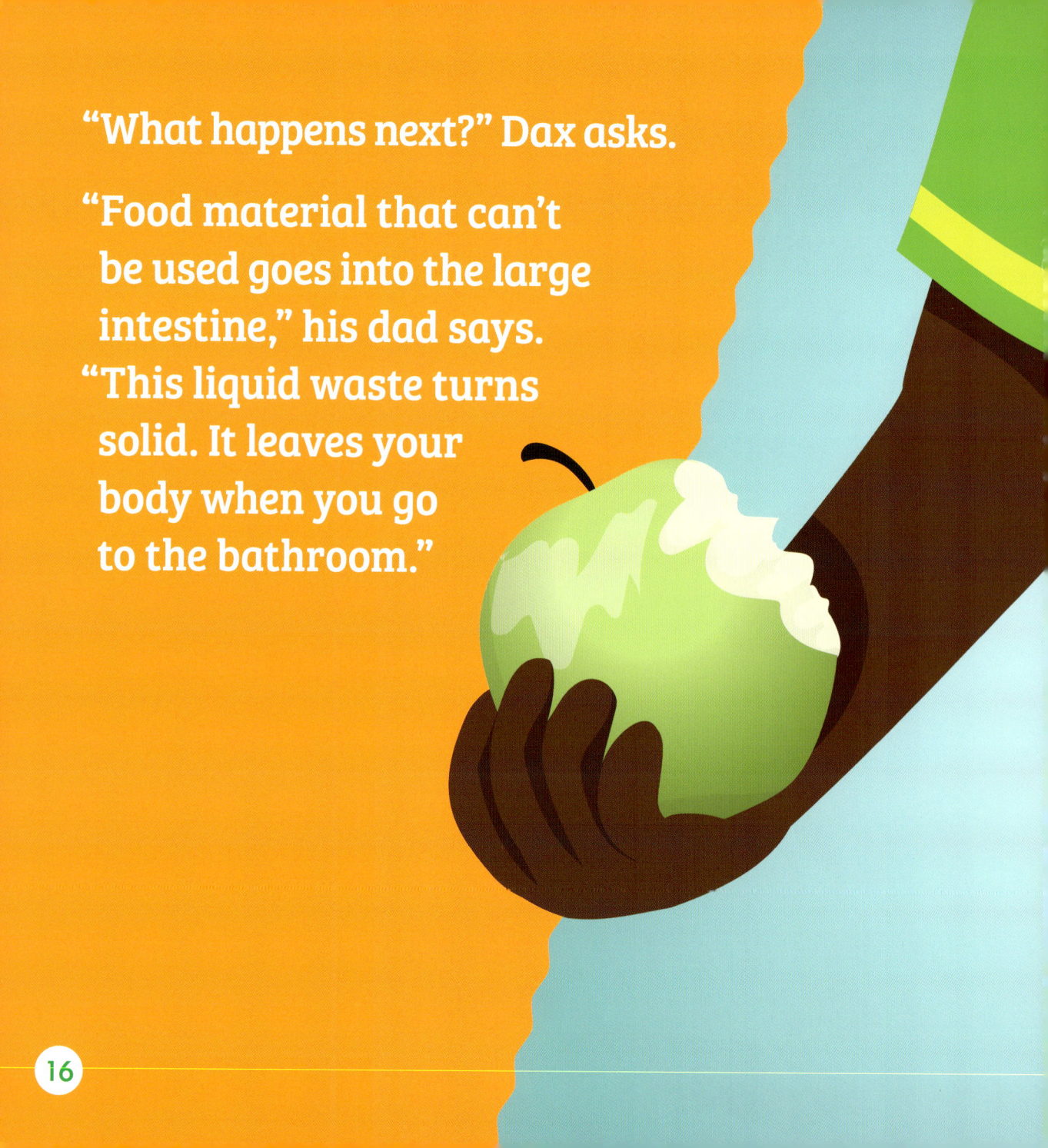

"Food material that can't be used goes into the large intestine," his dad says. "This liquid waste turns solid. It leaves your body when you go to the bathroom."

waste

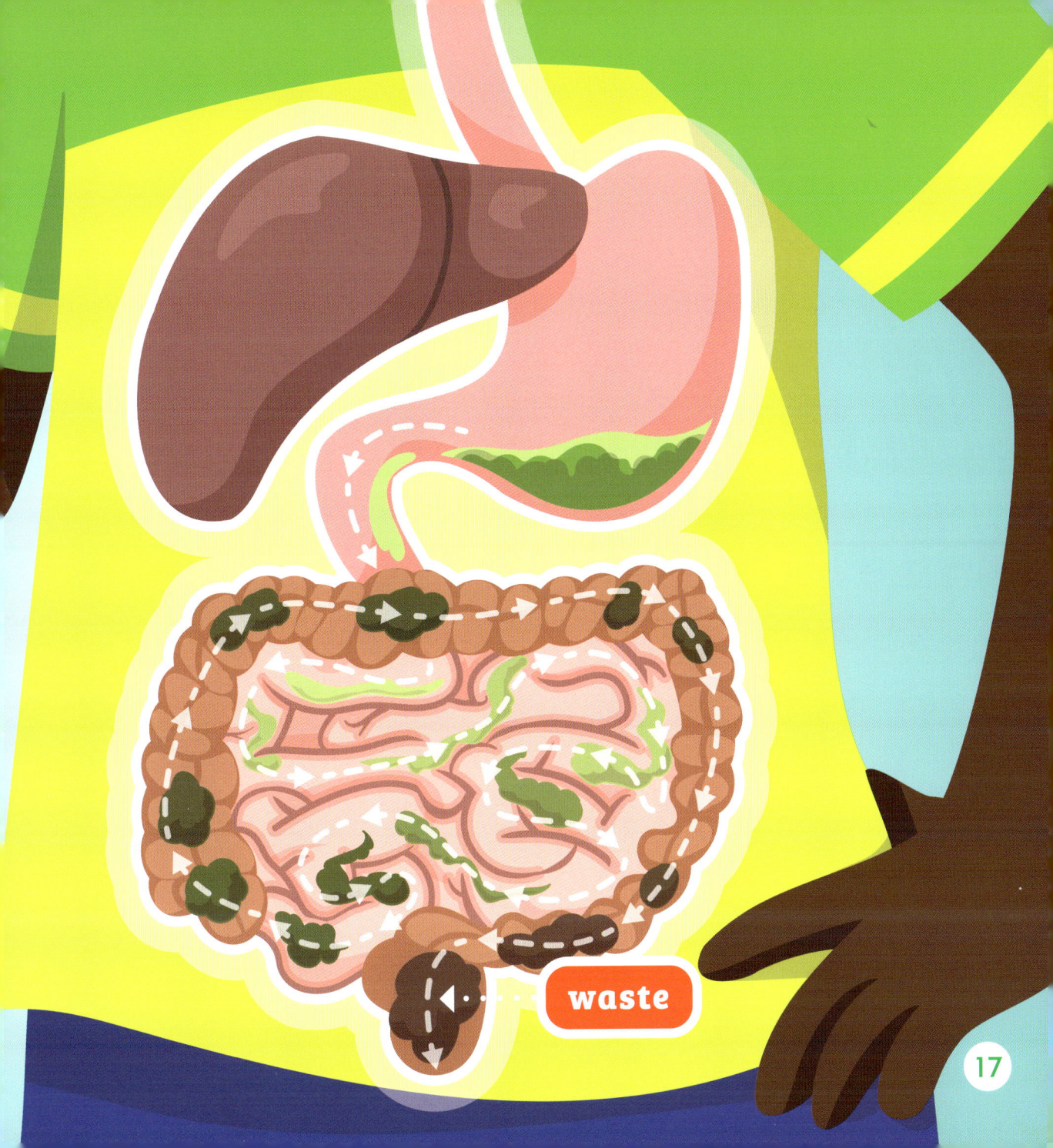

"So my digestive system does all of that every time I eat?" asks Dax.

"Yep! The next time you eat, the process starts over again. We depend on our digestive systems every day," his dad says.

19

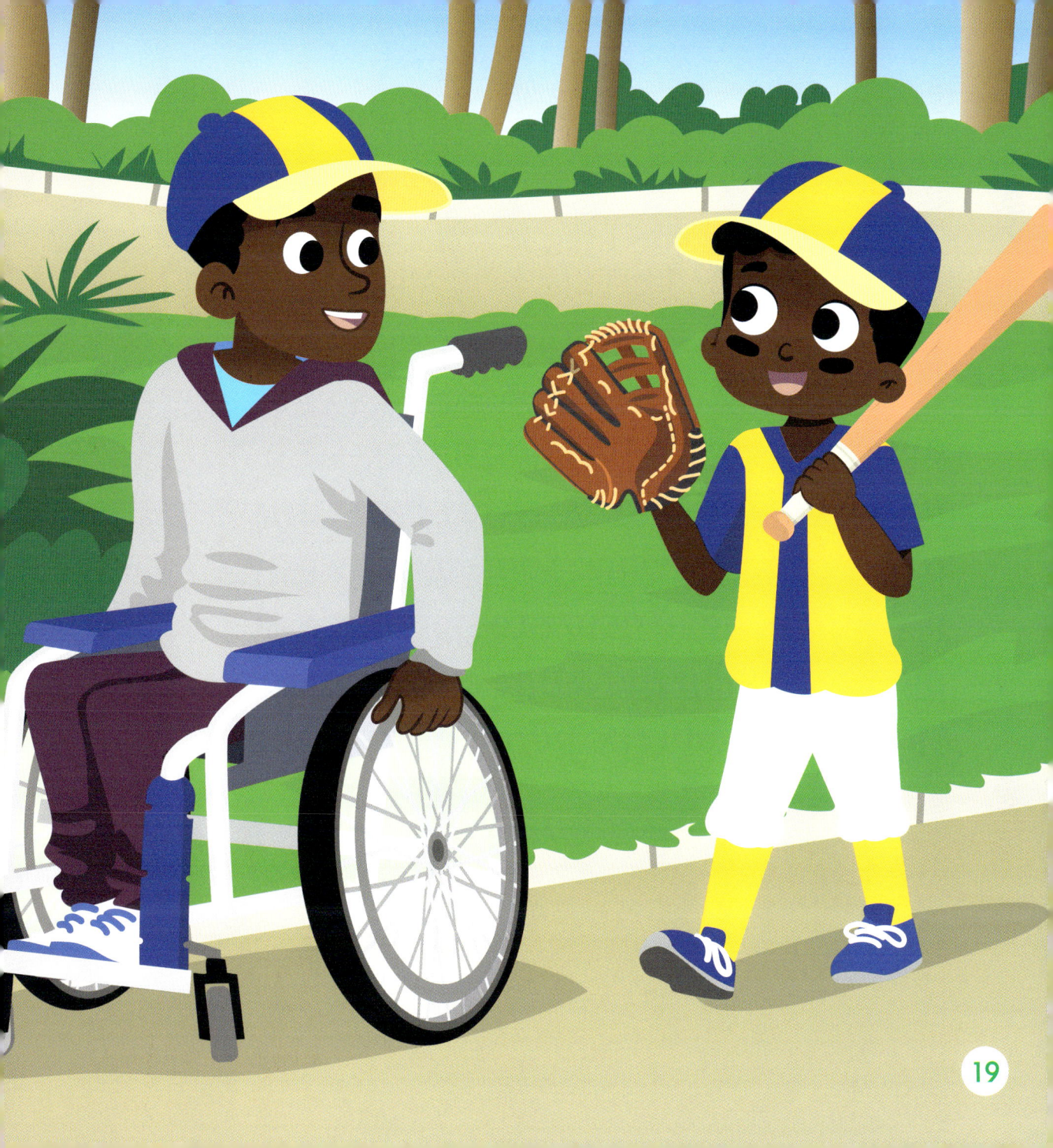

"Now go turn that energy from lunch into fuel for a home run!" Dax's dad says.

"Thanks, Dad! Cheer me on!" says Dax.

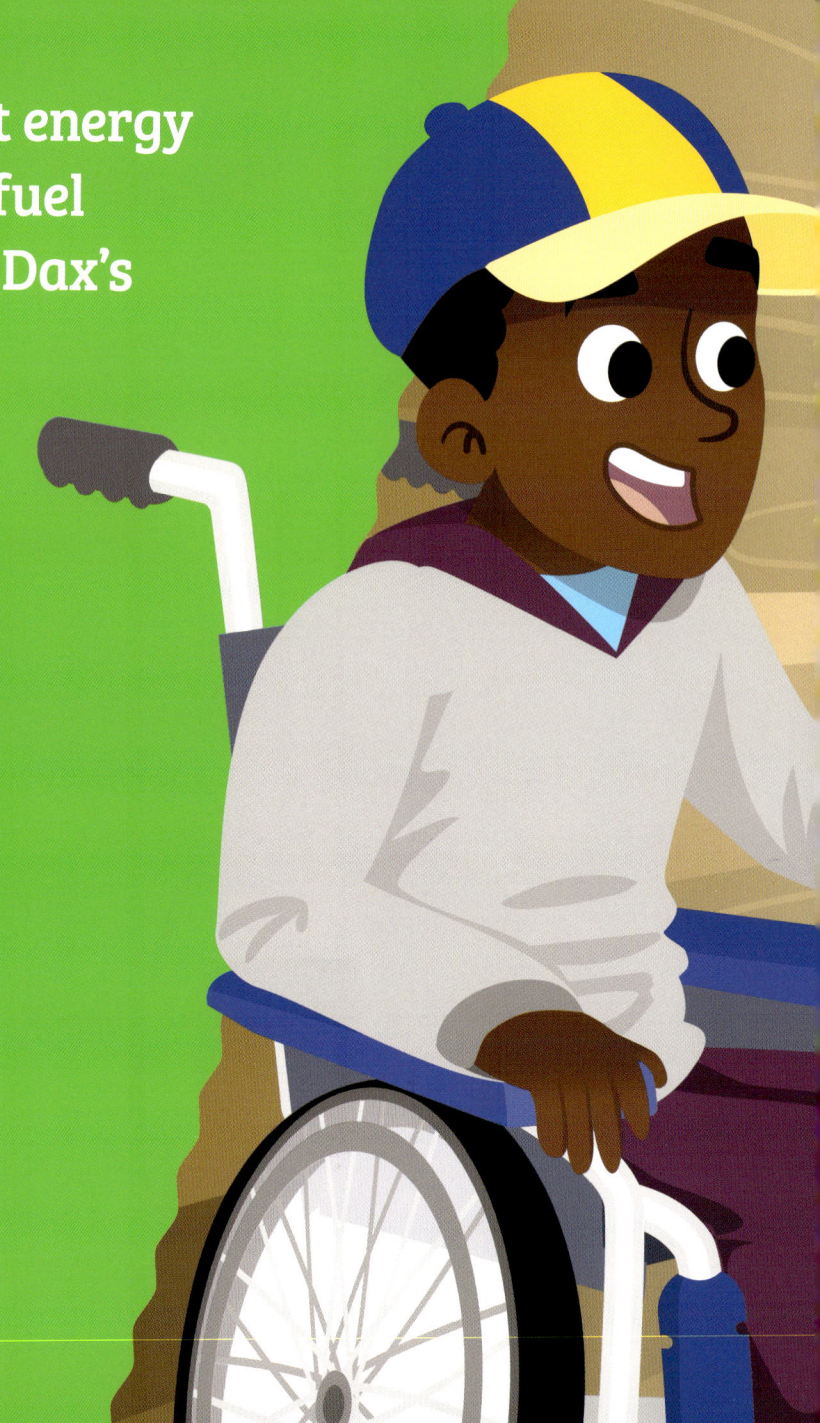

21

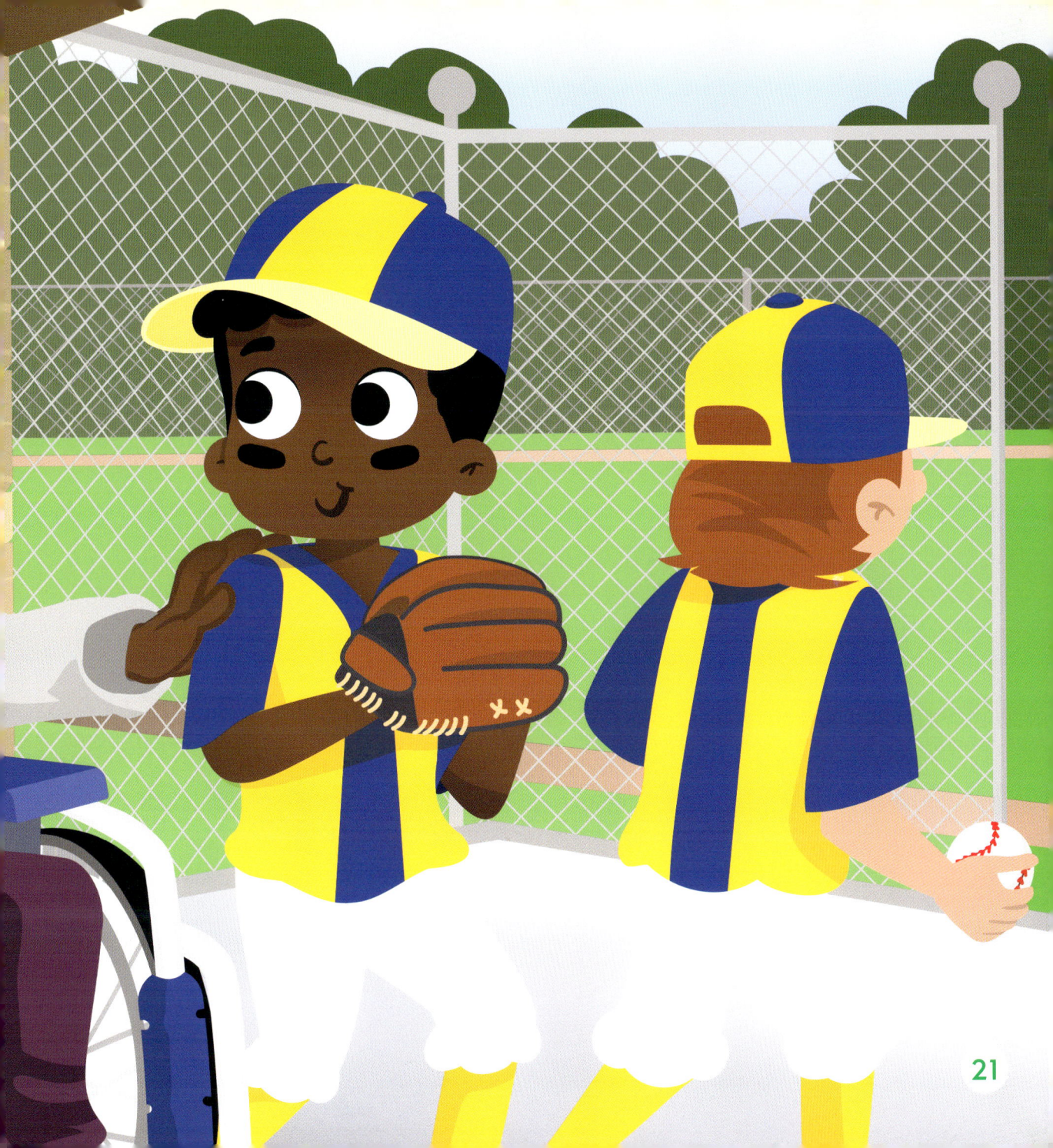

Where in the Body?

What are the major parts of the body's digestive system? Take a look!

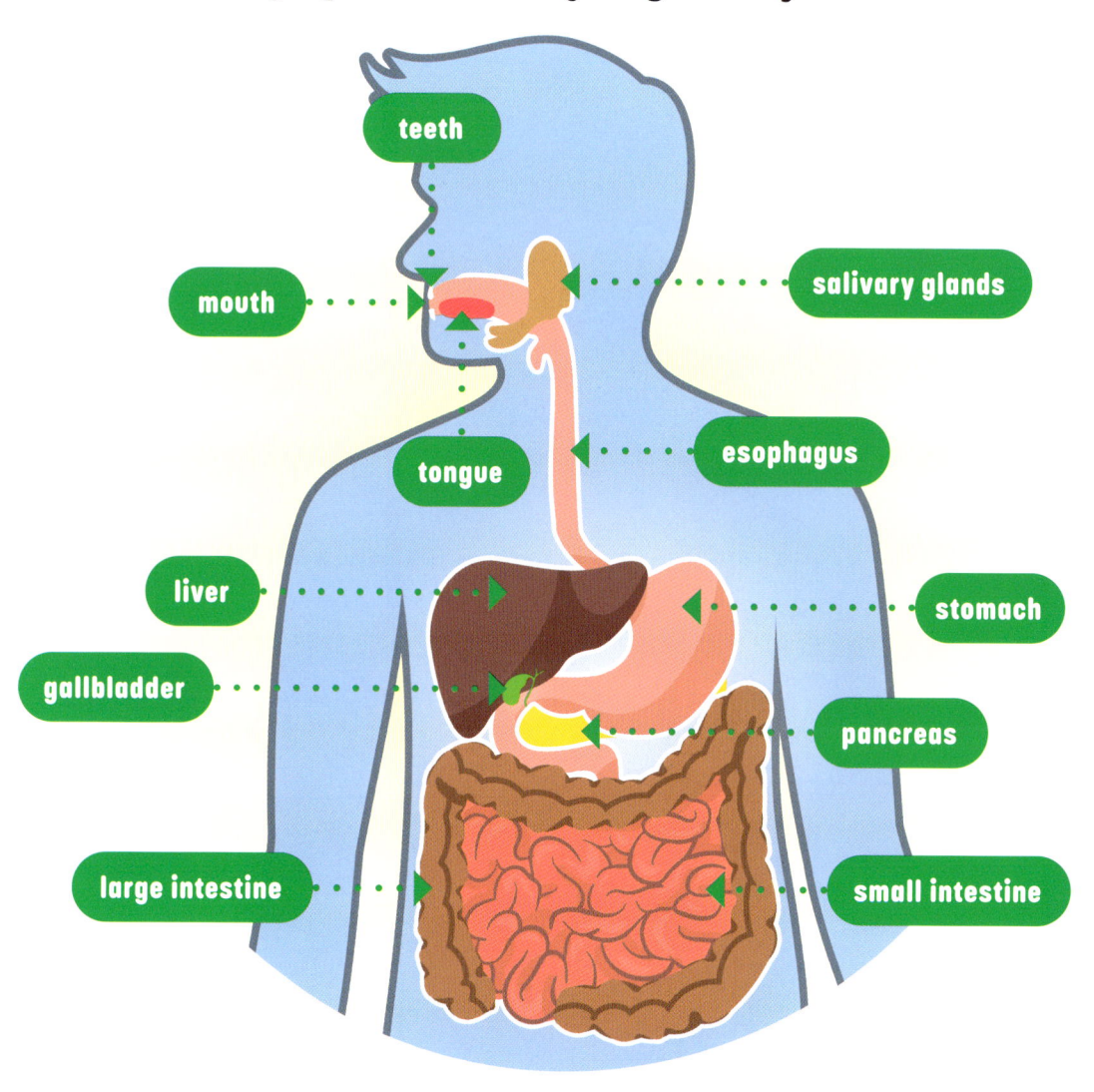

- teeth
- mouth
- salivary glands
- tongue
- esophagus
- liver
- stomach
- gallbladder
- pancreas
- large intestine
- small intestine

Let's Review!

The digestive system is made up of many organs. What three organs are shown here?

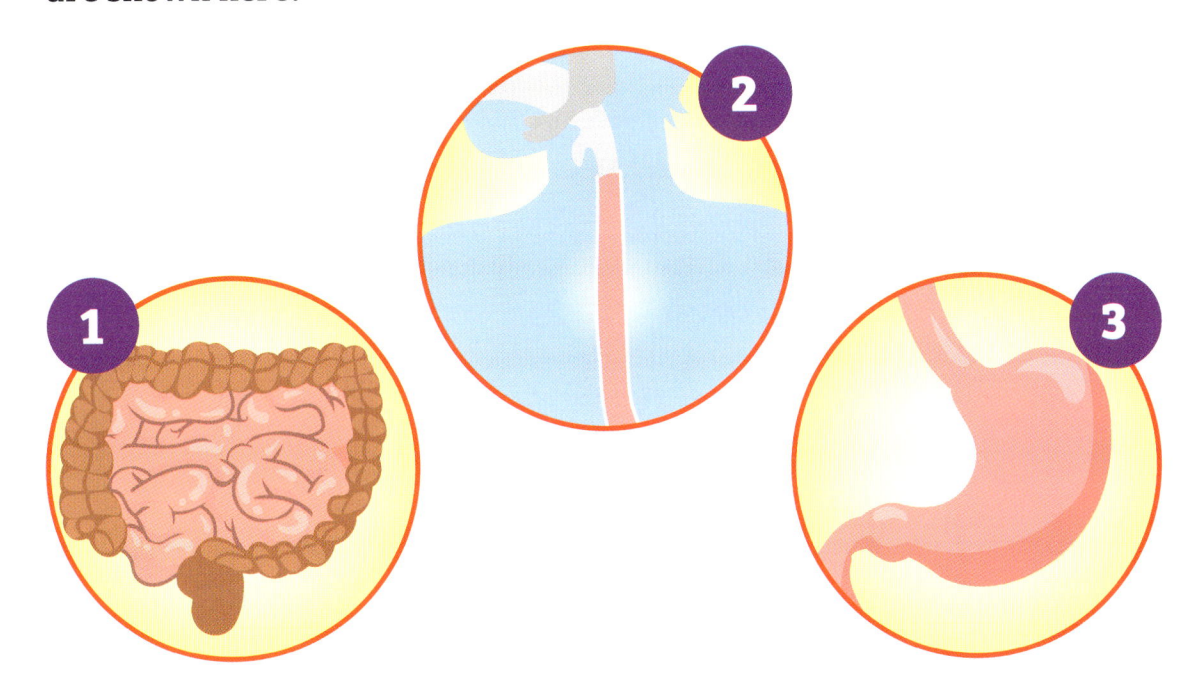

To Learn More

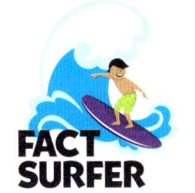

Finding more information is as easy as 1, 2, 3.

1. Go to www.factsurfer.com
2. Enter "**Dax'sdependabledigestivesystem**" into the search box.
3. Choose your book to see a list of websites.

Let's Review! Answer Key: **1.** intestines **2.** esophagus **3.** stomach

Glossary

acid: A liquid that can break food down.

cells: The smallest parts of living things. A microscope is needed to see cells.

digest: To break down food in the digestive organs so that it can be absorbed into the blood and used by the body.

energy: The strength to do things without getting tired.

enzymes: Proteins that help the body digest food.

hollow: Empty inside.

nutrients: Proteins, minerals, and vitamins your body needs to stay healthy and strong.

organs: Parts of the body that do certain jobs.

saliva: The watery fluid in your mouth that is secreted by glands and helps you soften and swallow food.

tissues: Masses of similar cells that form parts of organs.

Index

blood 14
digest 6
energy 6, 12, 14, 20
esophagus 9
food 5, 6, 8, 9, 10, 12, 15, 16
gallbladder 10
juices 10, 12
large intestine 16
liver 10

mouth 6
nutrients 6, 14, 15
pancreas 10
saliva 8
small intestine 14
stomach 4, 9, 12
teeth 8
tongue 8
waste 16